COMPLETE GUIDE TO LUNG TRANSPLANT

Essential Handbook To Surgery Procedures, Recovery Strategies, Risks & Benefits, Patient Success Stories, and Latest Medical Advances for Respiratory Health

DR. BRUNO HORAN

Disclaimer:

The information provided in this book, is intended for general informational purposes only and should not be considered as professional advice.

The author has made every effort to ensure the accuracy of the information presented. However, readers are advised to consult with a qualified healthcare professional before attempting any herbal remedies or making significant changes to their wellness routine. Individual health conditions vary, and what may be suitable for one person may not be appropriate for another.

It is important to note that the author is not in any endorsement deal, partnership, or affiliation with any organization, brand, or company mentioned in this book. Any references to specific products or services are based on the author's personal experience or general knowledge and do not imply an endorsement or promotion of those products or services

Contents

CHAPTER ONE 13

  PRE-TRANSPLANT EVALUATION 13

    Medical Assessments: Detailed Medical Tests And Screenings Are Required. 13

    Psychological Evaluation: Importance Of Mental Health Assessments. 14

    Lifestyle Changes: Necessary Lifestyle Adjustments Before Surgery...15

    Support System: Role Of Family And Caregivers In The Process. 16

    Financial Considerations: Understanding The Costs And Insurance Coverage...................................17

CHAPTER TWO 19

  FINDING A DONOR...19

    Donor Matching Process: How Donors And Recipients Are Matched 20

    Organ Allocation System: Understanding The Organ Allocation System..................................21

    Waiting List: What To Expect While On The Transplant Waiting List...22

CHAPTER THREE 25

THE TRANSPLANT SURGERY 25

Preparation For Surgery: Steps To Take Before
The Day Of Surgery..25

Surgical Procedure: Detailed Explanation Of The
Lung Transplant Surgery......................................26

Risks And Complications: Potential Risks And How
They Are Managed 27

Post-Surgery Care: Immediate Care After The
Surgery 28

Recovery Time: Expected Recovery Timeline And
Milestones 29

CHAPTER FOUR 31

POST-TRANSPLANT CARE 31

Medication Regimen: Essential Medications And
Their Management 31

Follow-Up Visits: Importance Of Regular Medical
Check-Ups 32

Monitoring For Rejection: Signs Of Organ Rejection
And Treatment..33

Rehabilitation: Role Of Physical Therapy In
Recovery 34

Long-Term Care: Managing Health In The Long-Term Post-Transplant 35

CHAPTER FIVE 37

LIFESTYLE ADJUSTMENTS 37

Diet And Nutrition: Nutritional Guidelines For Transplant Patients 37

Exercise And Physical Activity: Recommended Physical Activities 38

Mental Health: Importance Of Mental Well-Being And Support Groups 39

Avoiding Infections: Tips For Preventing Infections 40

Returning To Work: Guidelines For Resuming Work And Normal Activities 41

CHAPTER SIX 43

DEALING WITH COMPLICATIONS 43

Common Post-Transplant Complications 43

Chronic Rejection 44

Infections 45

Organ Function Monitoring.................................. 46

Emergency Situations 47

CHAPTER SEVEN 49

PSYCHOLOGICAL AND EMOTIONAL SUPPORT 49

Emotional Impact: Coping With The Emotional Aspects Of A Transplant 49

Support Groups: Benefits Of Joining Transplant Support Groups..50

Counseling Services: Importance Of Professional Counseling..50

Patient Stories: Inspirational Stories From Transplant Survivors..51

Building Resilience: Strategies For Building Mental Resilience 52

CHAPTER EIGHT 55

ADVANCES IN LUNG TRANSPLANTATION 55

Medical Innovations: Latest Advancements In Lung Transplant Techniques 56

Research And Clinical Trials: Ongoing Research And How To Get Involved 57

Future Prospects: Future Trends And Improvements In Lung Transplantation 58

Policy Changes: Recent Changes In Transplant Policies And Regulations 59

CHAPTER NINE 61

COMMON CONCERNS AND FAQS 61

What Is A Lung Transplant?................................61

Who Is Eligible For A Lung Transplant?..............61

Frequently Asked Questions: Answers To The Most Common Questions 63

Patient Rights: Understanding The Rights Of Transplant Patients 65

Support Resources: List Of Resources And Organizations For Support 66

ABOUT THIS BOOK

This comprehensive guide, "Lung Transplant," serves as a vital resource for individuals navigating the complex journey of lung transplantation. It begins by demystifying the procedure, defining what a lung transplant entails, and its profound impact on improving both quality of life and survival rates for patients facing severe respiratory challenges. Delving into its historical evolution, the book traces key milestones that have shaped modern transplant practices, providing context to the advancements and breakthroughs that have made this life-saving procedure possible today.

The importance of understanding eligibility criteria and the initial assessment process cannot be overstated. Through detailed medical and psychological evaluations, potential candidates gain insights into the rigorous standards required for transplantation readiness. Equally crucial are the lifestyle adjustments and support systems necessary before and after surgery, addressing not only the physical demands but also the emotional and financial considerations that accompany such a significant medical intervention.

Navigating the complex landscape of donor matching and organ allocation, the book illuminates the intricate processes that determine compatibility and facilitate the critical match between donor and recipient. It offers a compassionate exploration of ethical considerations surrounding organ donation, ensuring a nuanced perspective on the profound impact of these decisions.

The heart of the book lies in its comprehensive coverage of the transplant surgery itself—from meticulous preparation and the intricacies of the surgical procedure to managing potential risks and complications. Post-surgery care and long-term management strategies are equally prioritized, emphasizing the importance of medication adherence, rehabilitation, and ongoing medical monitoring to optimize recovery and sustain long-term health.

Beyond medical protocols, the guide embraces holistic wellness, offering practical advice on nutrition, exercise, mental health, and infection prevention. It empowers patients with the knowledge needed to navigate daily challenges, return to normal activities, and foster resilience through support groups and professional counseling services.

This book not only educates but also inspires, weaving in patient stories and highlighting medical innovations that promise to reshape the future of lung transplantation. By addressing common concerns, dispelling myths, and providing a wealth of resources, it equips readers with the tools to make informed decisions and embark on their transformative journey toward renewed health and vitality.

CHAPTER ONE

PRE-TRANSPLANT EVALUATION

Medical Assessments: Detailed Medical Tests And Screenings Are Required.

Before undergoing a lung transplant, thorough medical assessments are crucial to evaluate the patient's overall health and suitability for the procedure.

These assessments typically include a series of tests to assess lung function, cardiovascular health, and overall fitness for surgery.

Pulmonary function tests (PFTs) measure lung capacity and function, helping doctors determine the extent of lung disease and the need for transplantation. Imaging tests such as CT scans provide detailed images of the lungs, identifying any structural abnormalities or disease progression.

Blood tests are conducted to assess organ function and screen for infections or other conditions that could affect transplant outcomes. Additionally, cardiac evaluations, including electrocardiograms (ECGs) and echocardiograms, ensure that the heart can withstand the stress of surgery and recovery. These comprehensive assessments form the foundation for determining the patient's candidacy and preparing them for the transplantation process.

Psychological Evaluation: Importance Of Mental Health Assessments.

Beyond physical health, psychological evaluations are integral to the lung transplant evaluation process. These assessments aim to evaluate the patient's mental and emotional readiness for transplantation, as well as their ability to cope with the challenges of surgery and recovery.

Psychologists or psychiatrists assess factors such as stress management, coping mechanisms, and social support networks.

Addressing psychological health ensures that patients are mentally prepared for the potential outcomes of transplantation, including complications and lifestyle changes. It also helps identify any underlying mental health conditions that may require treatment before surgery. By assessing both physical and psychological factors, healthcare teams can optimize patient outcomes and support holistic well-being throughout the transplant journey.

Lifestyle Changes: Necessary Lifestyle Adjustments Before Surgery.

Preparing for a lung transplant involves significant lifestyle adjustments to optimize health and enhance transplant success. Patients are advised to maintain a balanced diet rich in nutrients to support overall health and immune function. Smoking cessation is critical, as smoking can exacerbate lung disease and complicate post-transplant recovery.

Regular physical activity is encouraged to improve cardiovascular fitness and overall strength, which can facilitate recovery and reduce complications after surgery. Additionally, patients may need to adjust their medication regimen and adhere strictly to prescribed treatments to stabilize their condition before transplantation.

Support System: Role Of Family And Caregivers In The Process.

The support system of family members, friends, and caregivers plays a crucial role in the lung transplant journey. Emotional and practical support from loved ones can significantly impact a patient's well-being and adherence to pre-transplant protocols.

Caregivers often assist with transportation to medical appointments, medication management, and providing emotional support during the evaluation process.

Family members and caregivers may also participate in educational sessions to understand the transplant procedure, potential risks, and post-transplant care requirements. Their involvement helps create a supportive environment that enhances the patient's overall experience and improves outcomes following transplantation.

Financial Considerations: Understanding The Costs And Insurance Coverage.

Navigating the financial aspects of lung transplantation requires careful consideration and planning. The costs associated with transplantation include pre-transplant evaluations, surgical procedures, hospitalization, post-operative care, and lifelong immunosuppressive medications. Patients and their families should explore insurance coverage options to understand what expenses are covered and any out-of-pocket costs they may incur.

Financial counselors or social workers can guide you in accessing financial assistance programs, navigating insurance policies, and exploring alternative funding sources.

Understanding the financial implications allows patients to make informed decisions about their healthcare and ensures that they can access necessary resources throughout the transplant process.

CHAPTER TWO

FINDING A DONOR

Finding a suitable donor for a lung transplant is a critical step in the process, often filled with anticipation and hope for patients awaiting transplantation. Donors can come from deceased individuals who have generously chosen to donate their organs or from living donors, typically family members or close friends who wish to contribute to their loved one's health journey.

For deceased donors, the process begins when a potential donor is identified, usually in a hospital setting where medical staff determine if the organs are viable for transplantation. Factors such as the donor's medical history, cause of death, and organ function are carefully assessed to ensure compatibility and safety for the recipient.

Living donors, on the other hand, undergo extensive medical evaluations to determine if they are suitable candidates. This involves comprehensive testing of lung function, overall health, and compatibility with the recipient. Living donation is a deeply personal decision and requires thorough consideration of both medical and ethical implications.

Donor Matching Process: How Donors And Recipients Are Matched

The donor matching process is a meticulous procedure designed to maximize the chances of a successful transplant. It begins with extensive testing and evaluation of both potential donors and recipients to ensure compatibility in terms of blood type, tissue type, and overall health status. This matching process is crucial to minimize the risk of rejection and optimize the transplant's long-term success.

Medical teams use sophisticated algorithms and databases to identify potential matches based on various factors, including the urgency of the recipient's condition, geographic proximity, and medical compatibility. Once a suitable match is identified, the transplant team notifies the recipient and begins preparations for the surgery.

Organ Allocation System: Understanding The Organ Allocation System

The organ allocation system is a complex framework designed to allocate organs fairly and efficiently to patients in need of transplantation.

In the United States, organ allocation is managed by the United Network for Organ Sharing (UNOS), which oversees a nationwide system that prioritizes patients based on medical urgency, waiting time, and other relevant factors.

Organs such as lungs are allocated based on a scoring system that takes into account the severity of the recipient's illness, the availability of donor organs, and the compatibility between donor and recipient.

This system aims to ensure that organs are distributed equitably while prioritizing those with the most urgent medical needs.

Waiting List: What To Expect While On The Transplant Waiting List

Being on the transplant waiting list can be a challenging and uncertain time for patients and their families. Once listed, patients await their turn based on the organ allocation system's criteria. The waiting period can vary widely depending on factors such as blood type, medical urgency, and the availability of suitable donors.

During this time, transplant candidates undergo regular medical evaluations to monitor their health status and readiness for surgery.

Patients need to maintain open communication with their transplant team, follow prescribed treatments, and stay prepared to go to the hospital at short notice when a suitable donor becomes available.

Living Donors: Possibility and considerations for living donors

Living donation for lung transplants is relatively rare compared to other organs like kidneys, but it remains an option for some patients. Living donors are typically close relatives or friends who undergo thorough medical evaluations to ensure their safety and compatibility with the recipient. This process involves detailed assessments of lung function, overall health, and psychological readiness.

Potential living donors must carefully consider the risks and benefits of donation, including the physical recovery process and potential long-term implications. The decision to become a living donor is deeply personal and involves comprehensive discussions with medical professionals, transplant coordinators, and loved ones.

Ethical Considerations: Ethical issues surrounding organ donation

Ethical considerations play a significant role in lung transplantation, particularly concerning organ donation and allocation. Issues such as informed consent, autonomy, and equity in access to transplantation services are carefully addressed throughout the process.

Medical teams prioritize patient welfare and ensure that both donors and recipients fully understand the implications of transplantation.

Ethical guidelines and legal frameworks help safeguard the rights of all parties involved, ensuring transparency, fairness, and respect for individual autonomy throughout the donation and transplantation process.

CHAPTER THREE

THE TRANSPLANT SURGERY

Preparation For Surgery: Steps To Take Before The Day Of Surgery

Preparing for a lung transplant surgery involves several crucial steps to ensure both physical readiness and logistical arrangements.

Initially, extensive medical evaluations will be conducted to assess overall health and suitability for transplantation.

This includes tests such as blood work, imaging scans, pulmonary function tests, and cardiac assessments to evaluate heart health.

Once cleared for surgery, patients are typically placed on a waiting list for donor lungs. During this waiting period, it's essential to maintain optimal health through prescribed medications, exercise routines tailored to individual capabilities, and adherence to dietary guidelines.

Patients are also advised to prepare emotionally and practically by organizing support networks for the recovery period and arranging for necessary accommodations during hospital stays.

Surgical Procedure: Detailed Explanation Of The Lung Transplant Surgery

Lung transplant surgery is a complex procedure performed under general anesthesia. The surgical team begins by making an incision in the chest to access the diseased lungs.

Depending on the type of transplant (single or double lung), the damaged lungs are carefully removed, making way for the donor lungs.

The new lungs are then meticulously attached to the pulmonary arteries, veins, and airways, ensuring proper blood flow and oxygenation.

Throughout the surgery, advanced monitoring equipment tracks vital signs to ensure stability. The procedure typically lasts several hours, during which the surgical team works with precision to minimize bleeding and optimize organ function. Post-surgery, chest tubes may be inserted to drain fluids and facilitate lung expansion.

Risks And Complications: Potential Risks And How They Are Managed

While lung transplant surgery offers hope for improved quality of life, it also carries risks. Common complications include infections, bleeding, blood clots, and rejection of the donor's lungs by the recipient's immune system.

To mitigate these risks, patients receive immunosuppressive medications to prevent rejection and antibiotics to prevent infections.

Close monitoring by healthcare professionals is crucial during the initial recovery phase to detect and address any complications promptly.

Post-Surgery Care: Immediate Care After The Surgery

Immediately following lung transplant surgery, patients are closely monitored in the intensive care unit (ICU). Ventilator support may be provided initially to assist with breathing until the new lungs begin functioning effectively.

Pain management is carefully administered to ensure comfort while avoiding complications. Physical therapy and respiratory exercises commence early to prevent complications such as pneumonia and promote lung function.

Nutritional support is also critical, with dietary adjustments tailored to support healing and immune function.

Regular medical assessments monitor organ function, medication levels, and signs of rejection or infection. Family and caregivers play a vital role in providing emotional support and assisting with daily activities during the recovery period.

Recovery Time: Expected Recovery Timeline And Milestones

Recovery from lung transplant surgery varies among individuals but generally follows a structured timeline. In the immediate post-surgery phase, patients remain in the hospital for several weeks under close medical supervision.

Gradually, as lung function improves and complications are managed, patients may transition to a rehabilitation facility or return home with outpatient monitoring.

Over the following months, adherence to prescribed medications and rehabilitation programs is crucial for successful recovery.

Milestones such as improved breathing capacity, reduced dependency on supplemental oxygen, and increased physical endurance signify progress. Long-term follow-up care continues to monitor lung function, manage medications, and address any emerging health concerns to optimize outcomes and quality of life.

CHAPTER FOUR

POST-TRANSPLANT CARE

After undergoing a lung transplant, diligent post-transplant care is crucial for ensuring a successful recovery and long-term health. This phase marks the beginning of a new chapter, where careful attention to medical guidelines and lifestyle adjustments can significantly impact your well-being.

Medication Regimen: Essential Medications And Their Management

Following a lung transplant, you will be prescribed a regimen of medications designed to prevent organ rejection and manage any potential complications. These medications typically include immunosuppressants to suppress the immune system's response, thereby reducing the risk of rejection. It's essential to adhere strictly to your medication schedule as prescribed by your healthcare team. Missing doses or altering the schedule without medical advice can compromise the success of your transplant.

In addition to immunosuppressants, other medications such as antibiotics, antifungals, and antivirals may be prescribed to prevent infections, which can be particularly concerning due to the immunosuppressed state post-transplant. Each medication plays a critical role in maintaining the health of your new lungs and managing any side effects or complications that may arise.

Follow-Up Visits: Importance Of Regular Medical Check-Ups

Regular follow-up visits with your transplant team are vital to monitor your progress, assess the function of your new lungs, and detect any signs of complications early. These visits allow your healthcare providers to adjust your medication regimen as needed, address any concerns you may have, and ensure that you are on track with your recovery.

During these visits, various tests such as pulmonary function tests, chest X-rays, and blood tests may be conducted to evaluate lung function and overall health.

Your transplant team will also guide lifestyle modifications, including diet and exercise recommendations tailored to support your recovery and long-term health.

Monitoring For Rejection: Signs Of Organ Rejection And Treatment

Despite diligent medication adherence, organ rejection can occur following a lung transplant. It's essential to be aware of the signs and symptoms of rejection, which may include shortness of breath, fever, fatigue, and decreased exercise tolerance.

If you experience any of these symptoms, it is crucial to notify your transplant team immediately.

Monitoring for rejection typically involves regular blood tests to measure the levels of immunosuppressants in your system and to detect any signs of rejection early.

Treatment for rejection may involve adjusting your medication regimen, increasing the dosage of immunosuppressants, or, in severe cases, hospitalization for intensive treatment.

Rehabilitation: Role Of Physical Therapy In Recovery

Physical therapy plays a crucial role in your recovery after a lung transplant. It helps improve lung function, strength, endurance, and overall mobility. Your transplant team will tailor a rehabilitation program to your individual needs, focusing on exercises to enhance breathing techniques, improve chest expansion, and build muscle strength.

Rehabilitation may begin shortly after surgery, starting with gentle exercises and gradually progressing as your strength and endurance improve. Your physical therapist will guide you through exercises both in the hospital and at home, providing instructions on proper techniques and monitoring your progress closely.

Long-Term Care: Managing Health In The Long-Term Post-Transplant

Long-term care following a lung transplant involves ongoing vigilance and commitment to maintaining your health.

This includes continuing with regular medical check-ups, adhering to your medication regimen, adopting a healthy lifestyle, and avoiding exposure to infections and environmental pollutants that could compromise lung function.

Your transplant team will guide managing chronic conditions, such as hypertension, diabetes, and osteoporosis, which may arise as a result of long-term immunosuppressant use.

They will also offer support and resources to help you navigate the challenges of life post-transplant, including emotional and psychological adjustments.

By prioritizing your health and following the recommendations of your transplant team, you can maximize the benefits of your lung transplant and enjoy a fulfilling life with improved respiratory function and overall well-being.

CHAPTER FIVE

LIFESTYLE ADJUSTMENTS

Diet And Nutrition: Nutritional Guidelines For Transplant Patients

Following a lung transplant, maintaining a healthy diet is crucial for recovery and long-term well-being. Transplant patients often require specific dietary adjustments to support their immune system and overall health. A balanced diet rich in fruits, vegetables, lean proteins, and whole grains helps in managing medications and preventing complications. It's important to monitor fluid intake and manage sodium levels to avoid fluid retention, which can strain the newly transplanted lungs.

Special attention should be given to food safety practices to prevent infections. This includes thoroughly washing fruits and vegetables, cooking meats thoroughly, and avoiding unpasteurized dairy products. It's recommended to work closely with a registered dietitian who can personalize nutritional recommendations based on individual needs and medication requirements. Regular follow-ups with healthcare providers help in adjusting dietary guidelines as recovery progresses.

Exercise And Physical Activity: Recommended Physical Activities

Physical activity plays a crucial role in recovery post-lung transplant. It helps in improving lung function, strengthening muscles, and maintaining overall cardiovascular health.

Initially, patients undergo supervised exercise programs tailored to their current health status and recovery phase. These programs gradually increase in intensity and duration as patients regain strength and endurance.

Recommended exercises include walking, light jogging, cycling, and swimming, depending on individual capabilities. Strength training exercises using resistance bands or light weights help in building muscle mass and enhancing stamina. It's important to avoid activities that pose a risk of injury or infection, such as contact sports or exposure to environmental pollutants. Regular monitoring by healthcare professionals ensures that exercise programs are safe and effective for each patient's recovery journey.

Mental Health: Importance Of Mental Well-Being And Support Groups

The emotional and psychological aspects of recovery after a lung transplant are significant. Patients may experience a range of emotions, including anxiety, stress, and depression, as they navigate the challenges of surgery and post-transplant care. It's crucial to prioritize mental well-being by seeking support from family, friends, and mental health professionals.

Joining support groups for transplant patients provides valuable peer support and practical advice on coping strategies. Engaging in relaxation techniques such as deep breathing exercises, meditation, or yoga can help reduce stress levels and promote emotional stability. Open communication with healthcare providers about emotional concerns ensures comprehensive care and timely interventions if needed.

Avoiding Infections: Tips For Preventing Infections

Preventing infections is a top priority for lung transplant recipients due to their weakened immune systems from anti-rejection medications. Simple precautions can significantly reduce the risk of infections. Patients should practice good hand hygiene by washing hands frequently with soap and water or using alcohol-based hand sanitizers.

Avoiding crowded places during flu season and wearing a mask in public settings further minimize exposure to respiratory viruses. It's essential to stay up-to-date with vaccinations recommended for transplant recipients, including annual flu shots and pneumonia vaccines. Maintaining a clean home environment, avoiding contact with sick individuals, and promptly reporting any signs of infection to healthcare providers are essential practices for infection prevention.

Returning To Work: Guidelines For Resuming Work And Normal Activities

Returning to work and normal activities after a lung transplant requires careful planning and coordination with healthcare providers. The timing of return varies depending on individual recovery progress, job requirements, and overall health status. Healthcare teams assess readiness based on physical stamina, immune system function, and ability to manage medications independently.

Patients are encouraged to start with part-time or modified work schedules initially to gradually build up stamina and adjust to work demands. Flexible work arrangements, such as telecommuting or modifying workstations for comfort and accessibility, support a smooth transition back to work. Open communication with employers about health needs and accommodations ensures a supportive work environment.

Regular follow-ups with healthcare providers monitor progress and address any challenges in resuming work activities. Patient education on recognizing signs of overexertion, managing fatigue, and balancing work with self-care routines enhances long-term success in maintaining employment post-transplant.

CHAPTER SIX

DEALING WITH COMPLICATIONS

Common Post-Transplant Complications

After a lung transplant, patients may experience various complications as their body adjusts to the new organ and immunosuppressive medications.

Common issues include infection, rejection, and side effects from medication. Infections are a significant concern due to the immunosuppressed state of the recipient, making them more vulnerable to bacterial, viral, and fungal infections.

These can affect the lungs or other parts of the body and require prompt treatment with antibiotics or antiviral medications.

Rejection occurs when the recipient's immune system recognizes the transplanted lung as foreign and tries to attack it. Acute rejection can happen within the first year post-transplant and is usually treatable with increased immunosuppression. Chronic rejection is a long-term concern where the body slowly damages the lungs over time, leading to decreased function. Monitoring for rejection involves regular lung function tests and biopsies to detect changes early.

Chronic Rejection

Chronic rejection, also known as chronic lung allograft dysfunction (CLAD), is a significant long-term complication post-lung transplant. It typically manifests as a progressive decline in lung function that is not reversible with treatment.

The exact cause of chronic rejection is not fully understood but is believed to involve both immune-mediated processes and non-immunologic factors.

Managing chronic rejection involves close monitoring of lung function through pulmonary function tests (PFTs) and imaging studies. Treatment options may include adjusting immunosuppressive medications to find the right balance between preventing rejection and minimizing side effects. In severe cases, re-transplantation may be considered if the decline in lung function is significant and irreversible.

Infections

Infections are a constant concern after lung transplantation due to the immunosuppressive medications that recipients must take to prevent rejection.

Types of infections can range from bacterial pneumonia to viral infections like cytomegalovirus (CMV) and fungal infections such as aspergillosis. Preventive measures include prophylactic antibiotics and antiviral medications, vaccination against certain infections before transplantation, and careful monitoring for symptoms.

Prompt recognition and treatment of infections are crucial to prevent complications such as pneumonia or sepsis. Lung transplant recipients are closely monitored for signs of infection during regular follow-up visits, and any suspected infection requires immediate medical evaluation and treatment.

Organ Function Monitoring

Monitoring the function of the transplanted lung is essential for detecting early signs of rejection or other complications. This involves regular pulmonary function tests (PFTs) to measure lung volumes and capacities, as well as spirometry to assess airflow. Imaging studies such as chest X-rays and CT scans help visualize the lung and detect any structural changes that may indicate rejection or infection.

Blood tests are also performed to monitor the levels of immunosuppressive medications and assess kidney function, as these medications can affect other organs over time.

Close collaboration between the transplant team and the patient is crucial to ensuring that any changes in organ function are promptly addressed to optimize long-term outcomes.

Emergency Situations

In emergencies post-lung transplant, prompt action is essential to ensure the best possible outcome. Emergencies may arise due to complications such as acute rejection, severe infection, or medication side effects.

Recognizing the signs of these complications early is key to initiating appropriate treatment and preventing further deterioration.

Patients are educated on symptoms that warrant immediate medical attention, such as sudden shortness of breath, chest pain, fever, or unexplained fatigue.

Transplant recipients need to have a plan in place for emergencies, including knowing whom to contact and where to go for specialized care. The transplant team guides managing emergencies and ensures that patients and caregivers are well-prepared to respond effectively.

CHAPTER SEVEN

PSYCHOLOGICAL AND EMOTIONAL SUPPORT

Emotional Impact: Coping With The Emotional Aspects Of A Transplant

Undergoing a lung transplant is a deeply emotional journey, impacting patients and their loved ones on various levels.

Emotions such as fear, anxiety, hope, and uncertainty are common throughout the process. Coping with these emotions is crucial for maintaining overall well-being and enhancing recovery outcomes.

Patients often experience a rollercoaster of feelings, from initial apprehension about surgery to hopefulness as they await a donor match. It's normal to feel overwhelmed or even elated at different stages.

Support Groups: Benefits Of Joining Transplant Support Groups

Transplant support groups provide invaluable emotional and practical support for patients undergoing lung transplants. These groups offer a safe space where individuals can share their experiences, fears, and successes with others who truly understand. Benefits include reducing feelings of isolation, gaining insights from fellow patients, and learning coping strategies from those who have walked a similar path. Support groups often foster a sense of community and camaraderie among members, which can significantly bolster morale during challenging times.

Counseling Services: Importance Of Professional Counseling

Professional counseling plays a pivotal role in helping lung transplant patients navigate the complex emotional landscape before, during, and after surgery.

Counselors provide a confidential environment where patients can express their fears, anxieties, and hopes openly. They offer tailored strategies to manage stress, enhance coping skills, and address any psychological barriers to recovery. Counseling sessions are designed to empower patients by equipping them with practical tools to handle emotional challenges effectively. This support is integral to promoting mental well-being and fostering resilience throughout the transplant journey.

Patient Stories: Inspirational Stories From Transplant Survivors

Listening to inspirational stories from lung transplant survivors can be incredibly uplifting and motivating for patients facing similar journeys. These stories highlight the resilience, courage, and determination of individuals who have overcome significant health challenges.

They offer hope and reassurance, showing that recovery is possible even in the face of adversity. Patient narratives also provide practical insights into coping strategies, medical milestones, and life post-transplant.

Hearing firsthand accounts of triumph over illness can inspire patients to stay positive and persevere through their recovery process.

Building Resilience: Strategies For Building Mental Resilience

Building mental resilience is essential for lung transplant patients as they navigate the ups and downs of their recovery journey.

Strategies include practicing mindfulness and relaxation techniques to reduce stress, maintaining a positive outlook by focusing on achievable goals and engaging in activities that promote emotional well-being.

Developing a support network of family, friends, and healthcare professionals also strengthens resilience by providing practical assistance and emotional encouragement.

Building resilience empowers patients to adapt to challenges, maintain hope, and ultimately achieve a better quality of life post-transplant.

CHAPTER EIGHT

ADVANCES IN LUNG TRANSPLANTATION

Lung transplantation has witnessed remarkable advancements in recent years, significantly improving outcomes and expanding eligibility criteria for patients with end-stage lung disease. One of the key advancements lies in surgical techniques, where minimally invasive approaches have become more prevalent.

These techniques reduce surgical trauma, minimize recovery times, and improve overall patient comfort post-transplantation.

Additionally, advancements in immunosuppressive therapies have enhanced long-term graft survival by effectively managing rejection while minimizing side effects.

Another critical advancement involves organ preservation methods. Innovations in organ perfusion technologies have extended the viability of donor lungs, allowing for better matching and reducing the risk of organ rejection. This has been complemented by improvements in donor selection criteria and the use of ex vivo lung perfusion (EVLP) to assess and rehabilitate marginal donor lungs, expanding the donor pool and increasing transplant opportunities.

Medical Innovations: Latest Advancements In Lung Transplant Techniques

Recent medical innovations in lung transplantation have revolutionized the field, offering new hope to patients suffering from severe lung diseases. One notable advancement is the development of personalized medicine approaches. Genetic testing and biomarker analysis now play a crucial role in tailoring immunosuppressive regimens, optimizing treatment outcomes, and reducing the risk of complications such as chronic rejection.

Moreover, advancements in surgical techniques have led to more precise and efficient procedures. Robotic-assisted surgery, for instance, allows for greater surgical precision and reduced recovery times compared to traditional open surgery. This approach benefits patients by minimizing trauma, enhancing postoperative recovery, and improving overall surgical outcomes.

Research And Clinical Trials: Ongoing Research And How To Get Involved

Ongoing research in lung transplantation focuses on several critical areas aimed at further improving patient outcomes and expanding treatment options. Clinical trials play a pivotal role in testing new therapies, surgical techniques, and innovative approaches to organ preservation and immunosuppression. Participating in clinical trials provides patients with access to cutting-edge treatments not yet widely available and contributes to advancing medical knowledge in the field.

Future Prospects: Future Trends And Improvements In Lung Transplantation

The future of lung transplantation holds promising prospects, driven by ongoing research and technological advancements. One of the anticipated trends is the development of bioengineered lungs using stem cell technology and 3D printing.

These approaches aim to create customized, patient-specific lungs that minimize the risk of rejection and offer long-term graft survival. Additionally, advances in artificial intelligence (AI) and machine learning are expected to enhance preoperative planning, organ matching, and postoperative care, further optimizing transplant outcomes.

Technological Developments: Role of Technology in Enhancing Outcomes

Technology continues to play a pivotal role in enhancing outcomes in lung transplantation. Advanced imaging techniques, such as high-resolution CT scans and positron emission tomography (PET), enable precise assessment of lung function and pathology before and after transplantation. This allows clinicians to monitor graft function closely, detect complications early, and tailor treatment strategies accordingly.

Policy Changes: Recent Changes In Transplant Policies And Regulations

Recent years have seen significant changes in transplant policies and regulations aimed at improving patient access, organ allocation fairness, and transplant outcomes.

Policy changes often focus on enhancing transparency in organ allocation processes, promoting equity in access to transplantation, and addressing ethical considerations in donor selection.

Additionally, regulatory updates ensure compliance with evolving standards of care, patient safety, and ethical guidelines in the field of lung transplantation.

CHAPTER NINE

COMMON CONCERNS AND FAQS

What Is A Lung Transplant?

A lung transplant is a surgical procedure where a diseased or failing lung is replaced with a healthy lung from a donor. It is typically considered when other treatments for severe lung conditions have been exhausted and the patient's quality of life is significantly impacted. The goal is to improve breathing and overall lung function, enabling the patient to lead a more active and fulfilling life.

Who Is Eligible For A Lung Transplant?

Eligibility for a lung transplant depends on several factors, including the severity of the lung condition, overall health, and the ability to undergo surgery and recovery. Patients are evaluated by a transplant team which includes specialists such as pulmonologists, surgeons, and social workers. Factors such as age, overall health, and the presence of other medical conditions are carefully assessed to determine suitability for transplantation.

What Conditions Can Require a Lung Transplant?

Conditions that may necessitate a lung transplant include chronic obstructive pulmonary disease (COPD), cystic fibrosis, pulmonary fibrosis, and severe pulmonary hypertension, among others. These conditions can severely limit lung function and quality of life despite medical management.

How is Lung Transplant Surgery Performed?

During a lung transplant surgery, the patient is placed under general anesthesia. The surgeon removes the diseased lung(s) and replaces them with healthy donor lung(s). The procedure can involve one lung (single lung transplant) or both lungs (double lung transplant), depending on the patient's condition and the recommendation of the transplant team.

What is the Recovery Process Like?

Recovery from a lung transplant surgery varies from patient to patient but generally involves several weeks in the hospital followed by a period of outpatient rehabilitation and monitoring. Medications to prevent organ rejection are crucial during this time, and patients will have regular follow-up appointments with their transplant team to monitor their progress and adjust treatment as needed.

Frequently Asked Questions: Answers To The Most Common Questions

How Long Does a Lung Transplant Surgery Take?

The duration of a lung transplant surgery can vary depending on the complexity of the case, but it typically ranges from four to twelve hours. Factors such as whether it's a single or double lung transplant and any unforeseen complications can affect the length of the procedure.

What are the Risks Associated with Lung Transplant Surgery?

Like any major surgery, lung transplant surgery carries risks such as infection, bleeding, organ rejection, and complications related to anesthesia. The transplant team works closely with each patient to minimize these risks through careful pre-operative preparation and post-operative care.

How Long Does it Take to Recover from a Lung Transplant?

Recovery time can vary, but most patients spend about two to three weeks in the hospital following surgery. Full recovery, including returning to normal activities, can take several months to a year or longer, depending on individual health and the progress of rehabilitation.

Myths and Facts: Dispelling Common Myths about Lung Transplants

Myth: Lung Transplants are Only for Young Patients.

Fact: Age alone does not disqualify someone from receiving a lung transplant. The decision is based on overall health and the ability to tolerate surgery and recovery.

Myth: Lung Transplants Always Require a Lifetime of Immunosuppressive Drugs.

Fact: While lifelong immunosuppressive therapy is often necessary to prevent rejection, advances in medicine have improved drug regimens and management, reducing side effects and improving outcomes.

Patient Rights: Understanding The Rights Of Transplant Patients

Patient Rights in the Transplant Process

Patients undergoing lung transplants have certain rights, including the right to be informed about their treatment options, the right to privacy and confidentiality, and the right to participate in decisions about their care. Understanding these rights helps ensure that patients receive the best possible care and support throughout the transplant journey.

Support Resources: List Of Resources And Organizations For Support

Organizations and Support Groups

Several organizations and support groups specialize in providing information, resources, and emotional support to lung transplant patients and their families. These include national transplant organizations, local support groups, and online communities where patients can connect with others who have undergone similar experiences.

Contact Information: Key Contacts for Further Information and Assistance

Transplant Centers and Hotlines

For further information about lung transplants, including eligibility criteria, surgery details, and support resources, patients and their families can contact transplant centers directly. Many centers also have dedicated hotlines staffed by transplant coordinators who can provide guidance and answer questions.